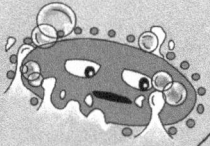
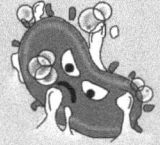

WASH EM DOWN COLORING BOOK

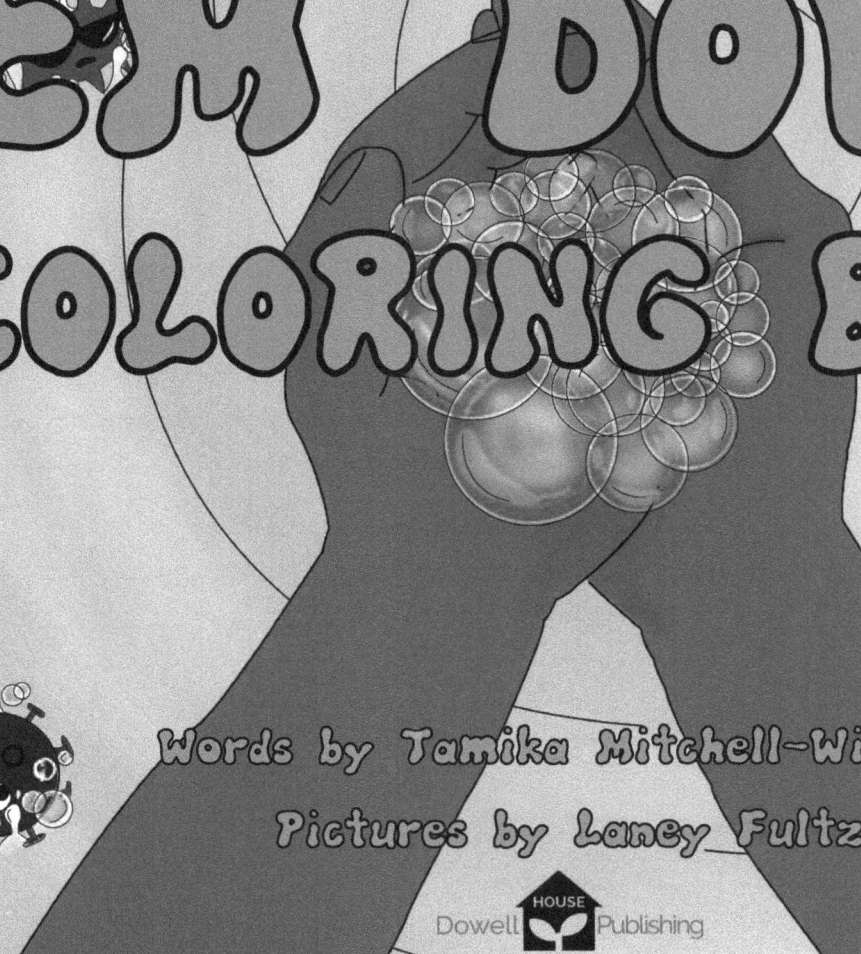
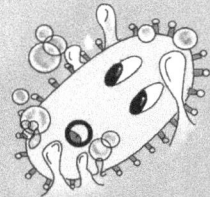
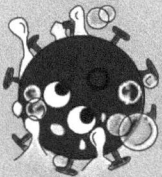

Words by Tamika Mitchell-Wilcher

Pictures by Laney Fultz

Dowell HOUSE Publishing

Dowell House Publishing, LLC
2221 Hampstead Dr.
Columbus, OH 43229
www.dowellhousepublishing.com

Original Wash "Em Down" book with color.
ISBN: 979-8-9858200-1-0
Library of Congress #: 2022914308

Illustrations by Laney Fultz
Digital and Graphic Editing: Ashley E. Dowell
Photography by Tamika Mitchell-Wilcher

Printed in the United States of America

Disclaimer:

The words in this book are intended to be a comedic parody of the song **Walk Em Down by NLE Choppa. The words in this book have not been professionally recorded by Tamika Wilcher to the tune of "Walk Em Down" and are not being sold for profit as a musical single. For an example of how you can match the words with the tune "Walk Em Down," please visit Tamika Wilcher's social media channels for much "cleaner" and more educational versions of the original songs!

Sing along with the "Wash Em Down" book here: https://www.youtube.com/watch?v=69-pxB2htE0

Check out her other social media pages for more songs and content!

TikTok: @educatedauthor3
Youtube: Teacher T's World

**Walk Em Down ©2020 NLE Choppa Entertainment Inc., under exclusive license to Warner Records Inc.

Music Notes PNGs by Vecteezy..com

WASH EM DOWN

COLORING BOOK

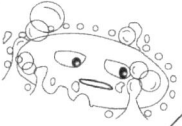

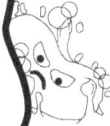

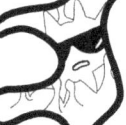

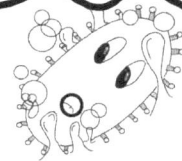

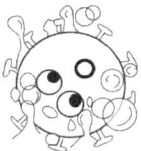

Posted in front of the sink.

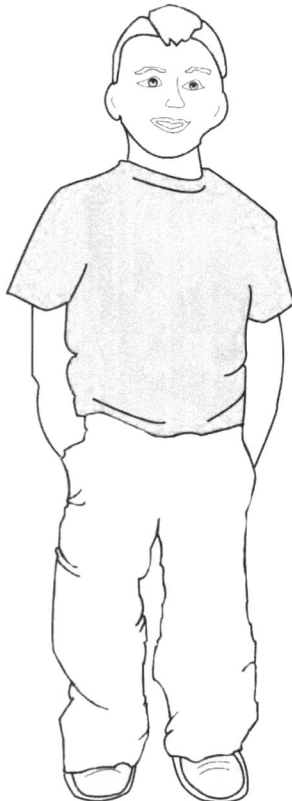

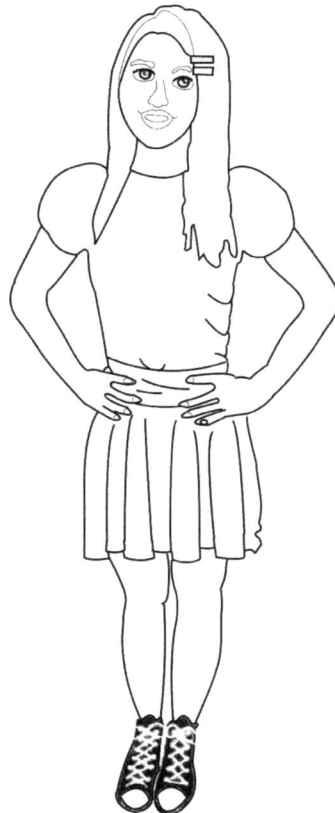

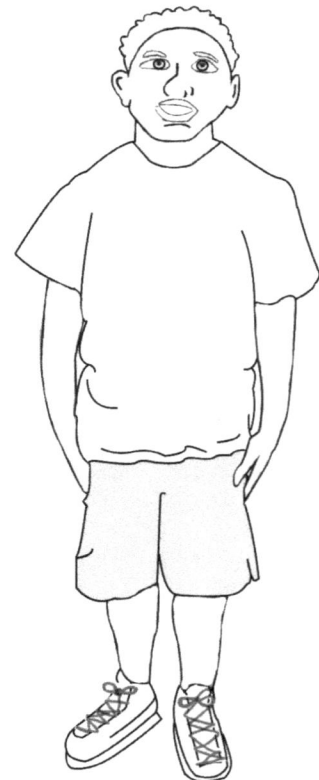

Getting ready to watch

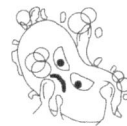

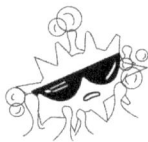

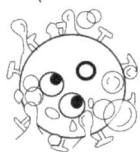

them germs go down!

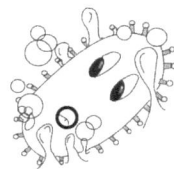

Turn on the tap
and apply the soap!

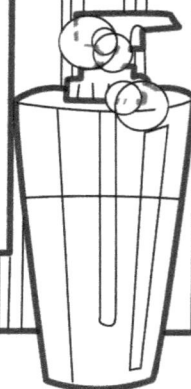

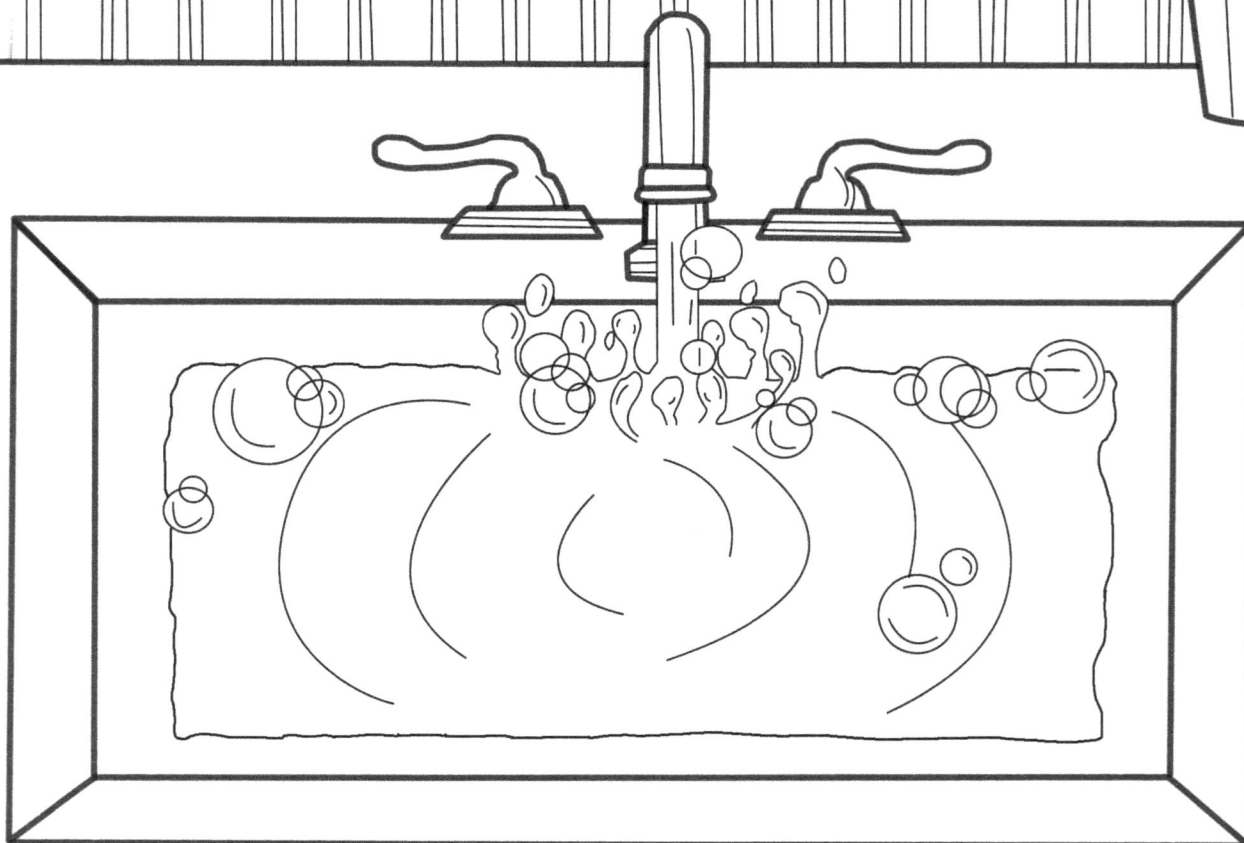

Then we make the hands go

round and round.

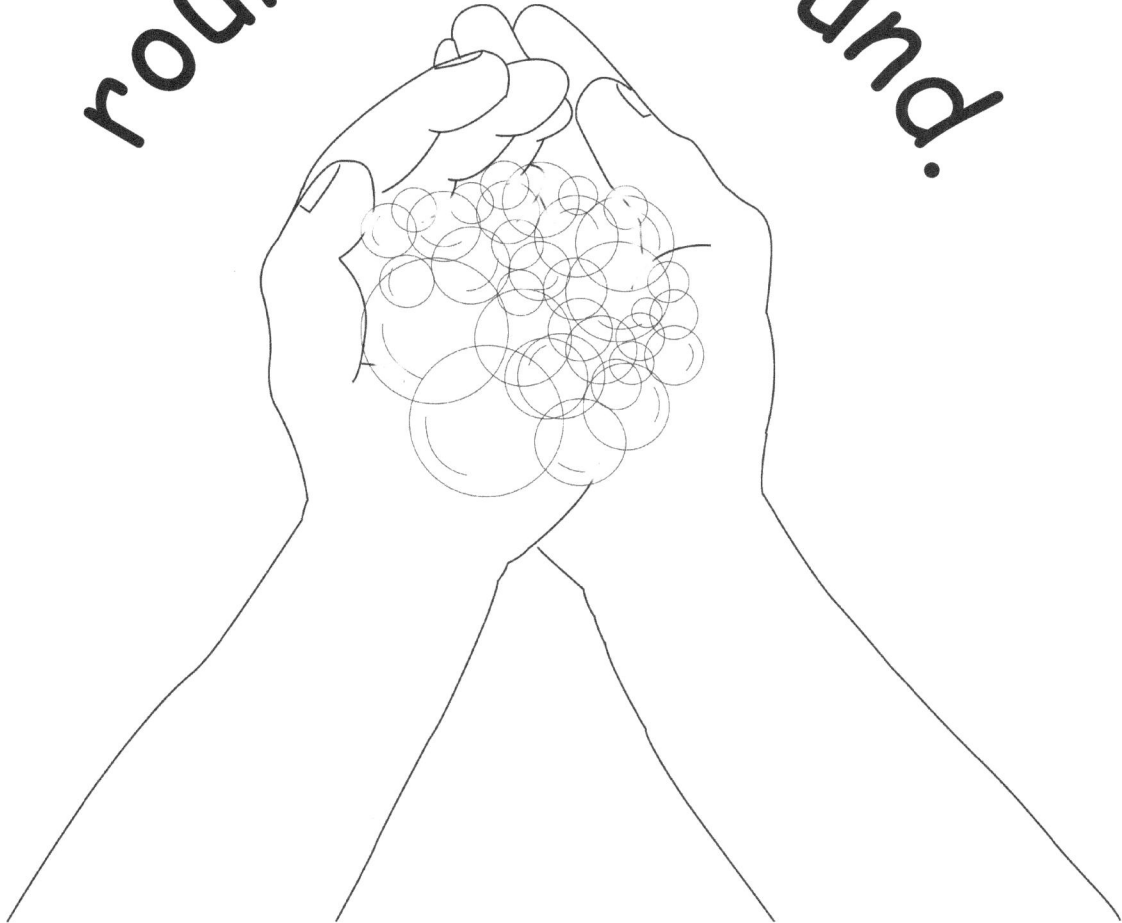

4

Aa Bb Cc Dd Ee Ff Gg Hh Ii

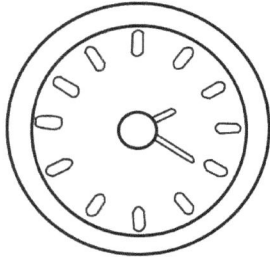

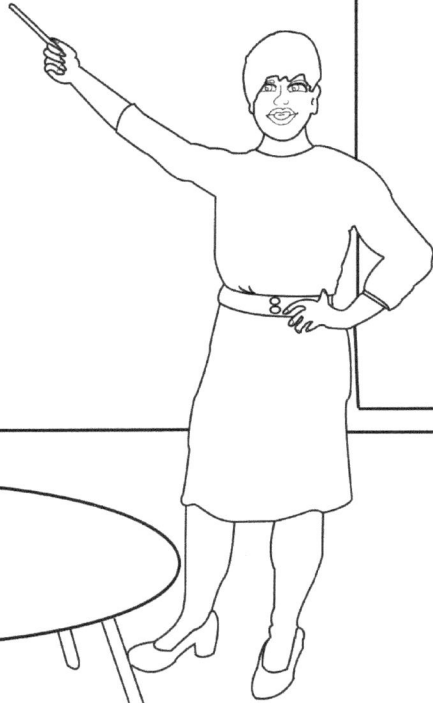

Teachers in the back with the clock.

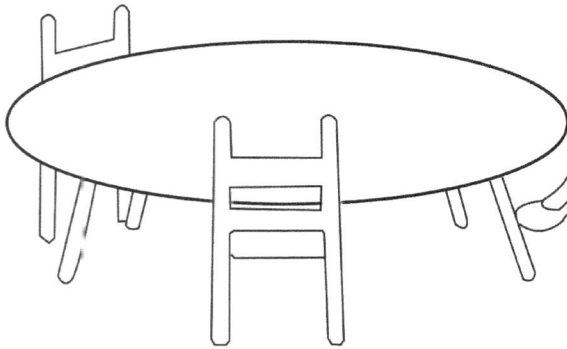

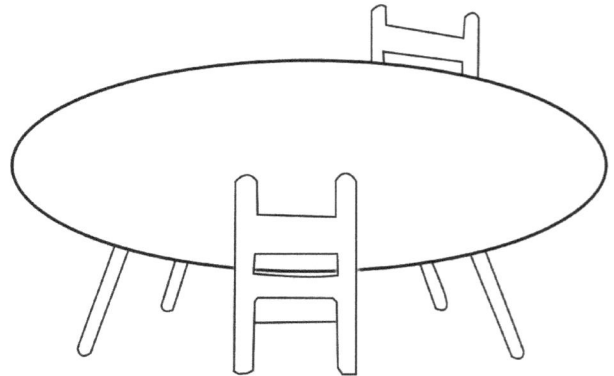

We got 20 seconds to make them germs go down.

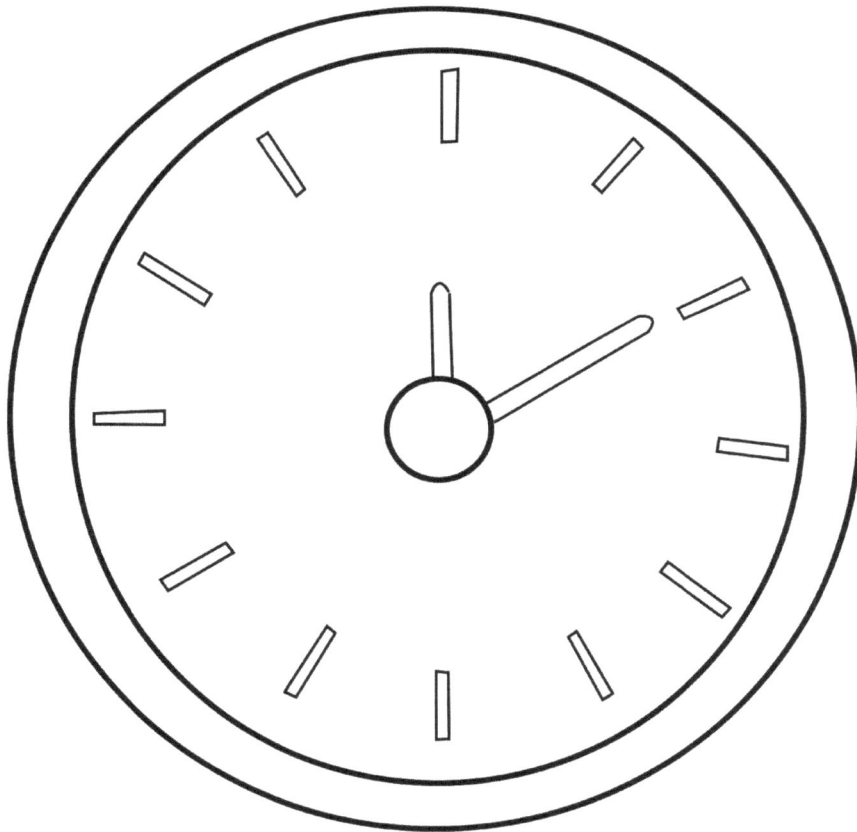

You think we hesitating 'cause she ain't playin'.

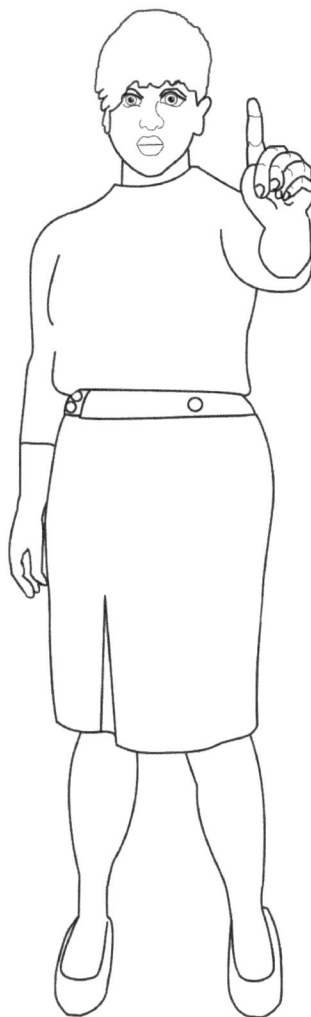

She **DON'T** like them germs
and we can't let her down.

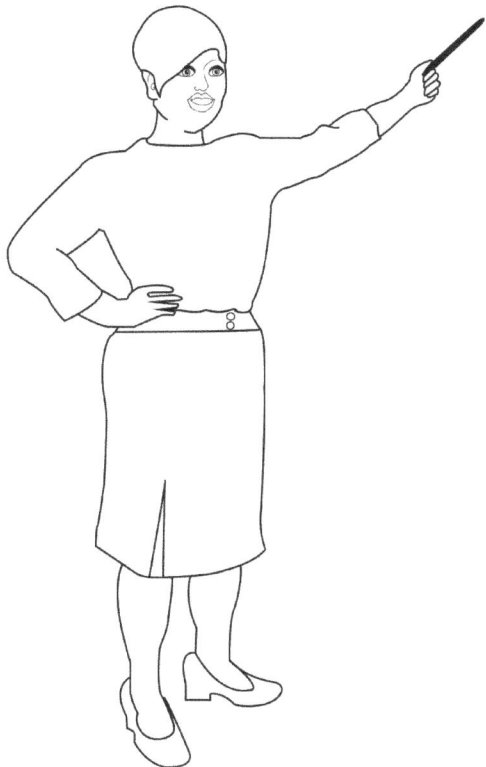

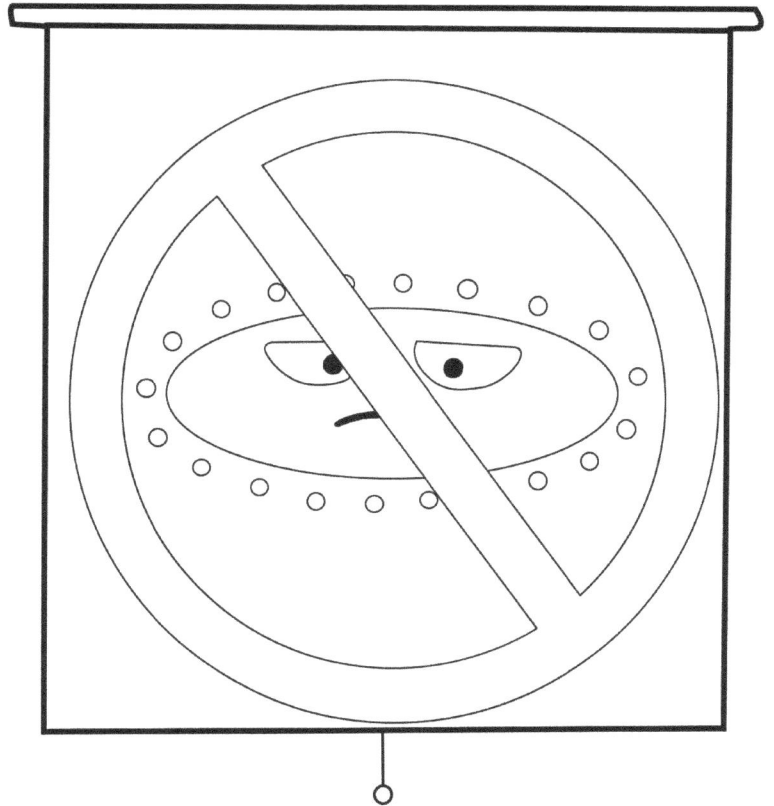

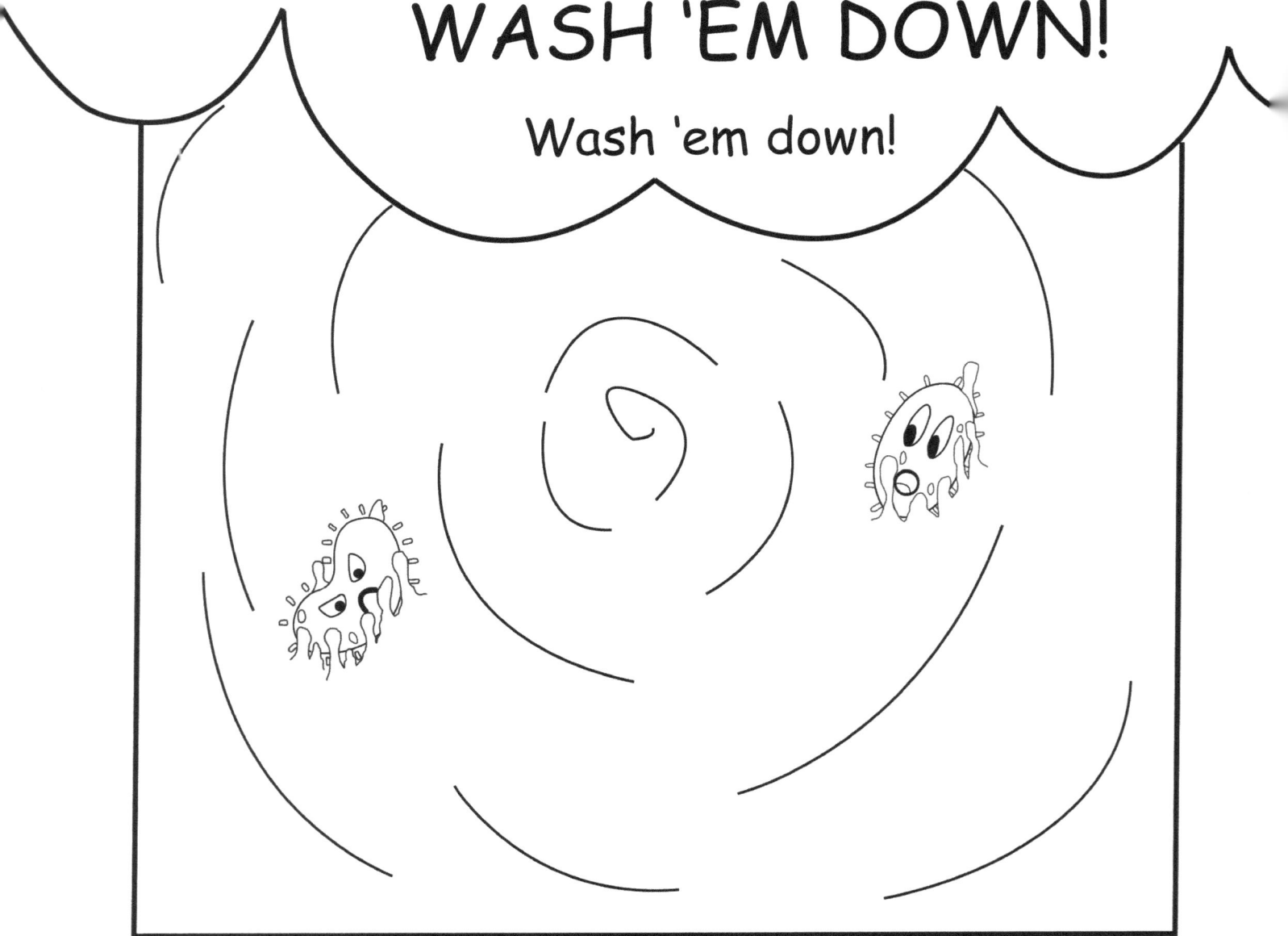

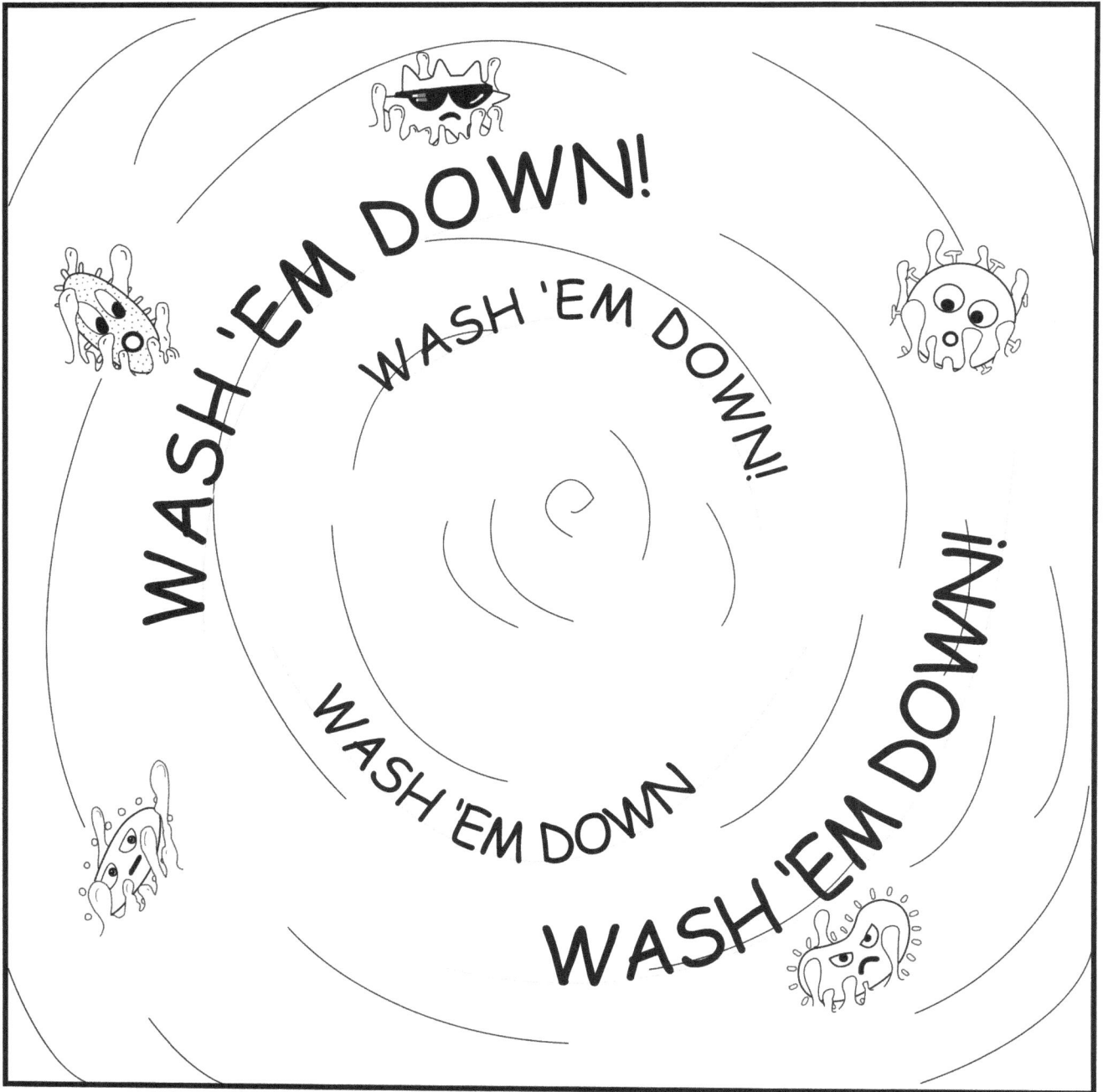

Look down on 'em while they runnin' down with water.

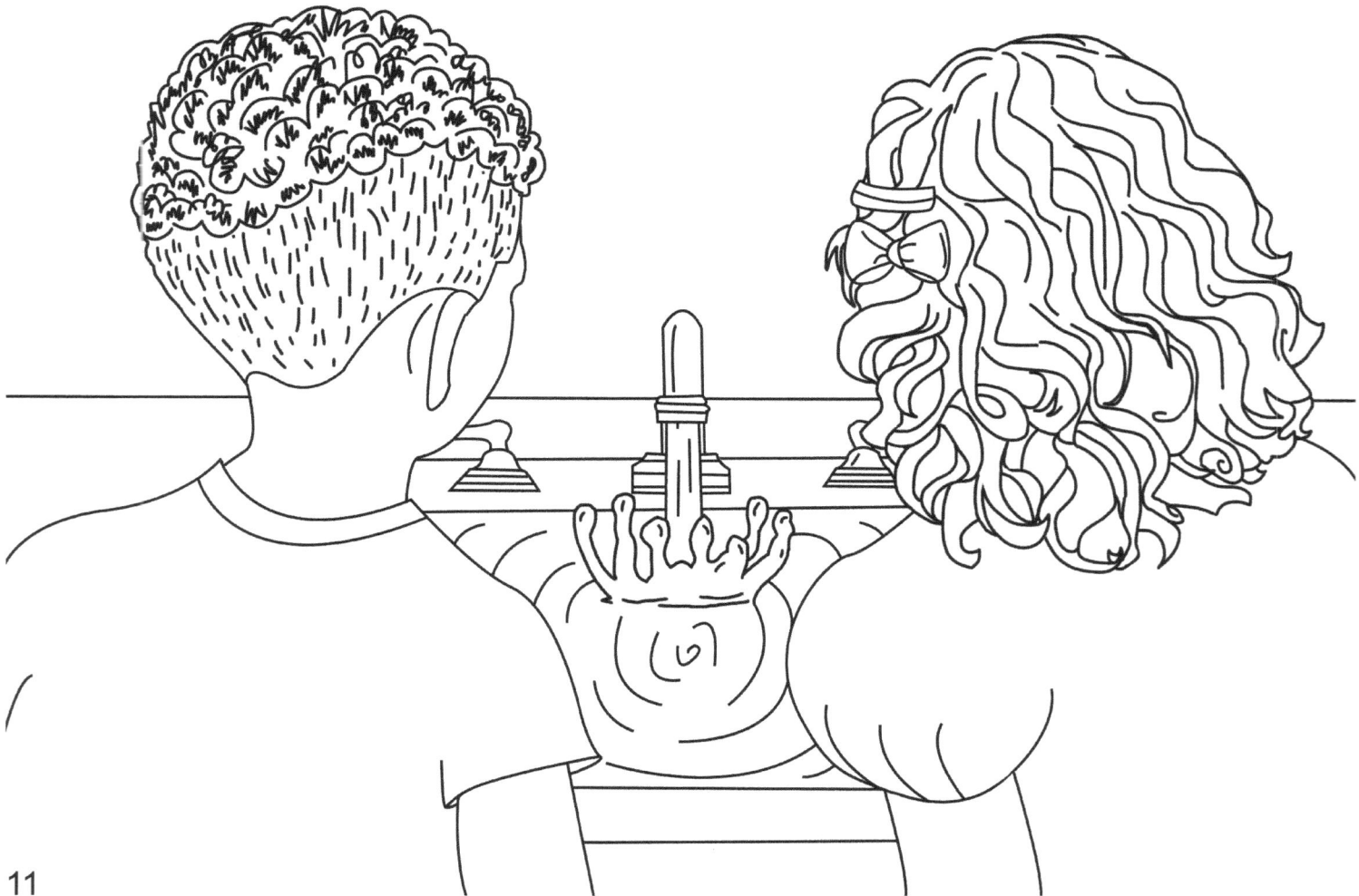

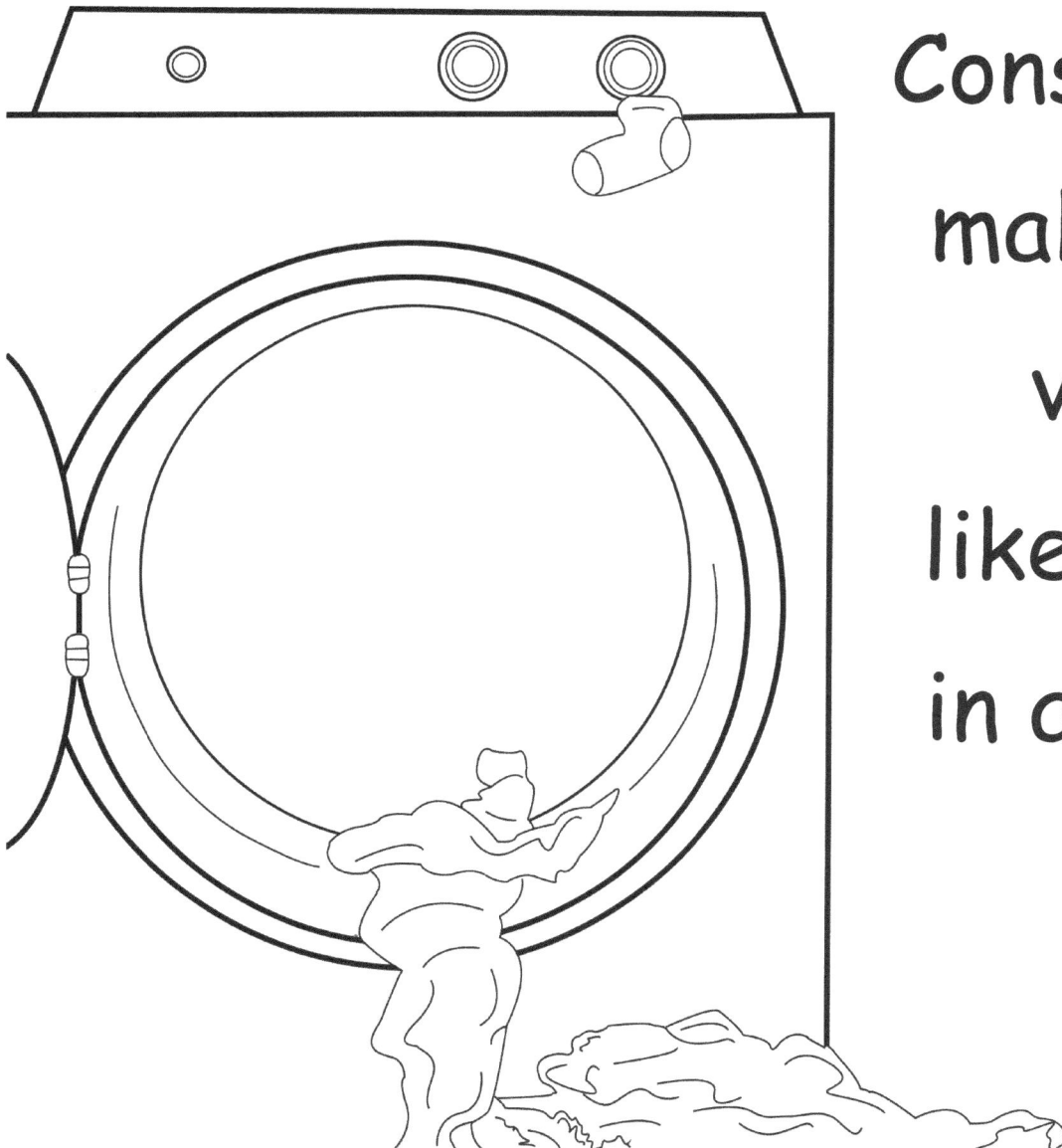

Consistency
makes 'em
vanish
like a sock
in a dryer.

You go against then you suck

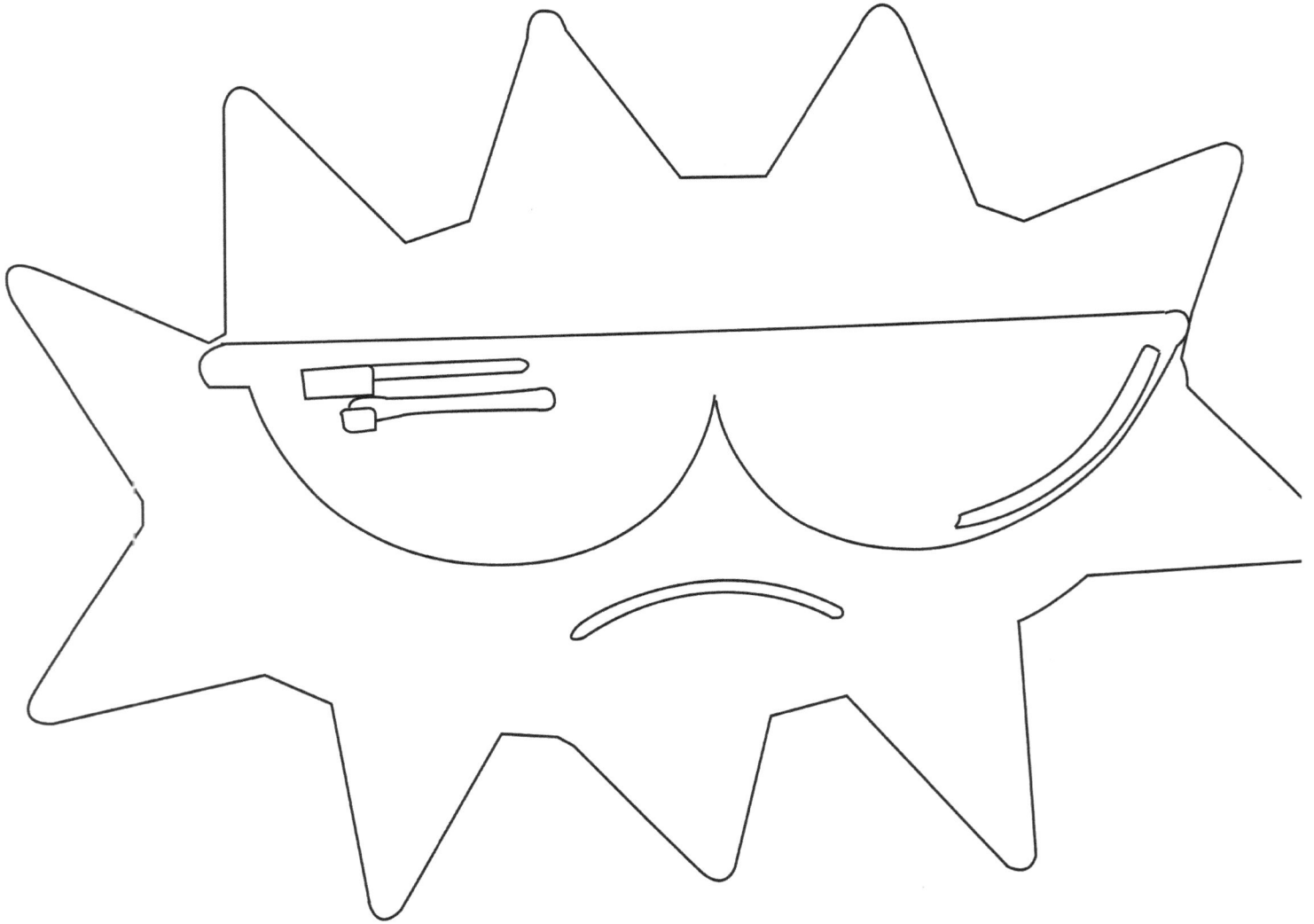

just like Coronavirus

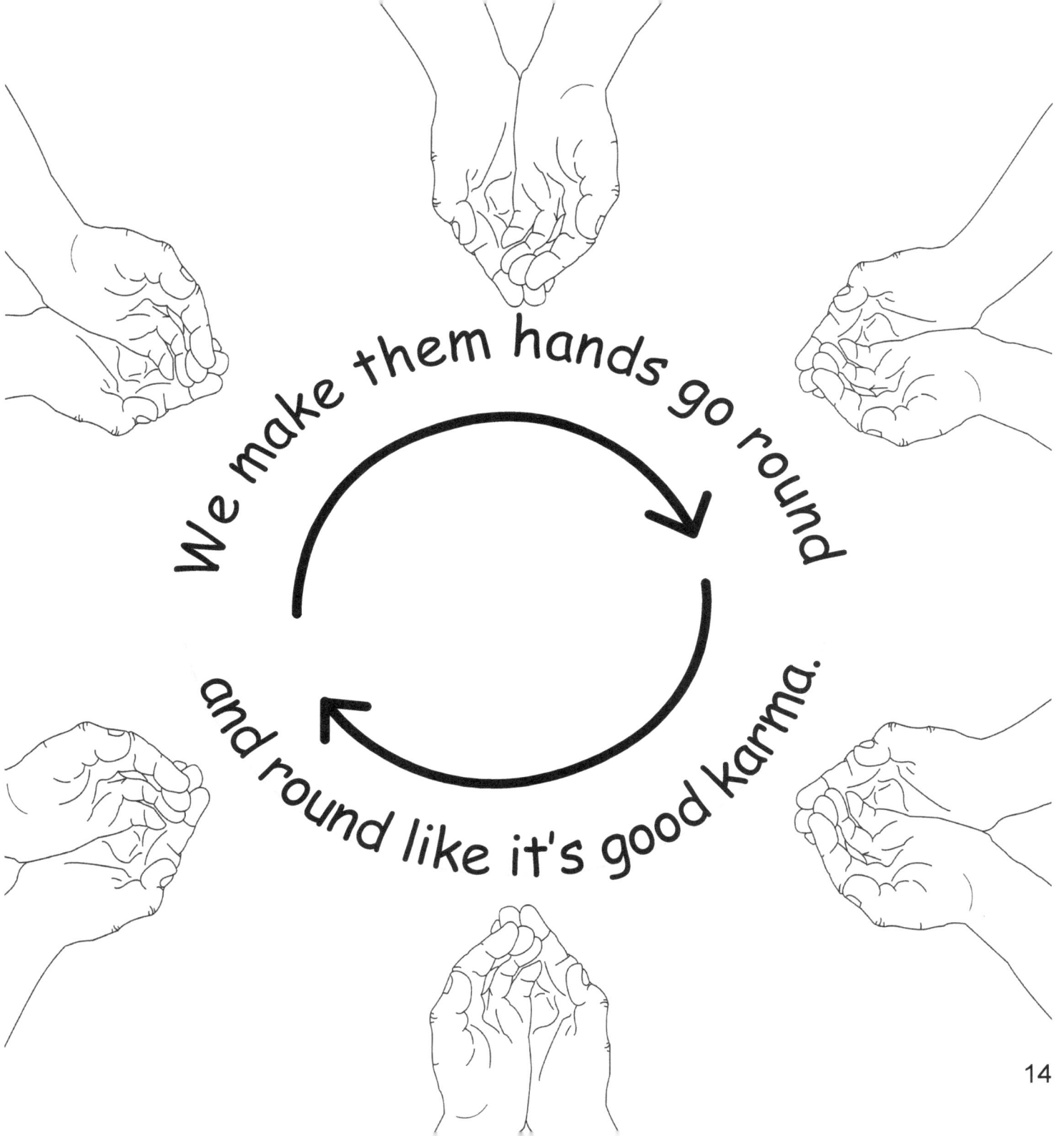

We make them hands go round and round like it's good karma.

They look really clean now,
but I wanna wash 'em.

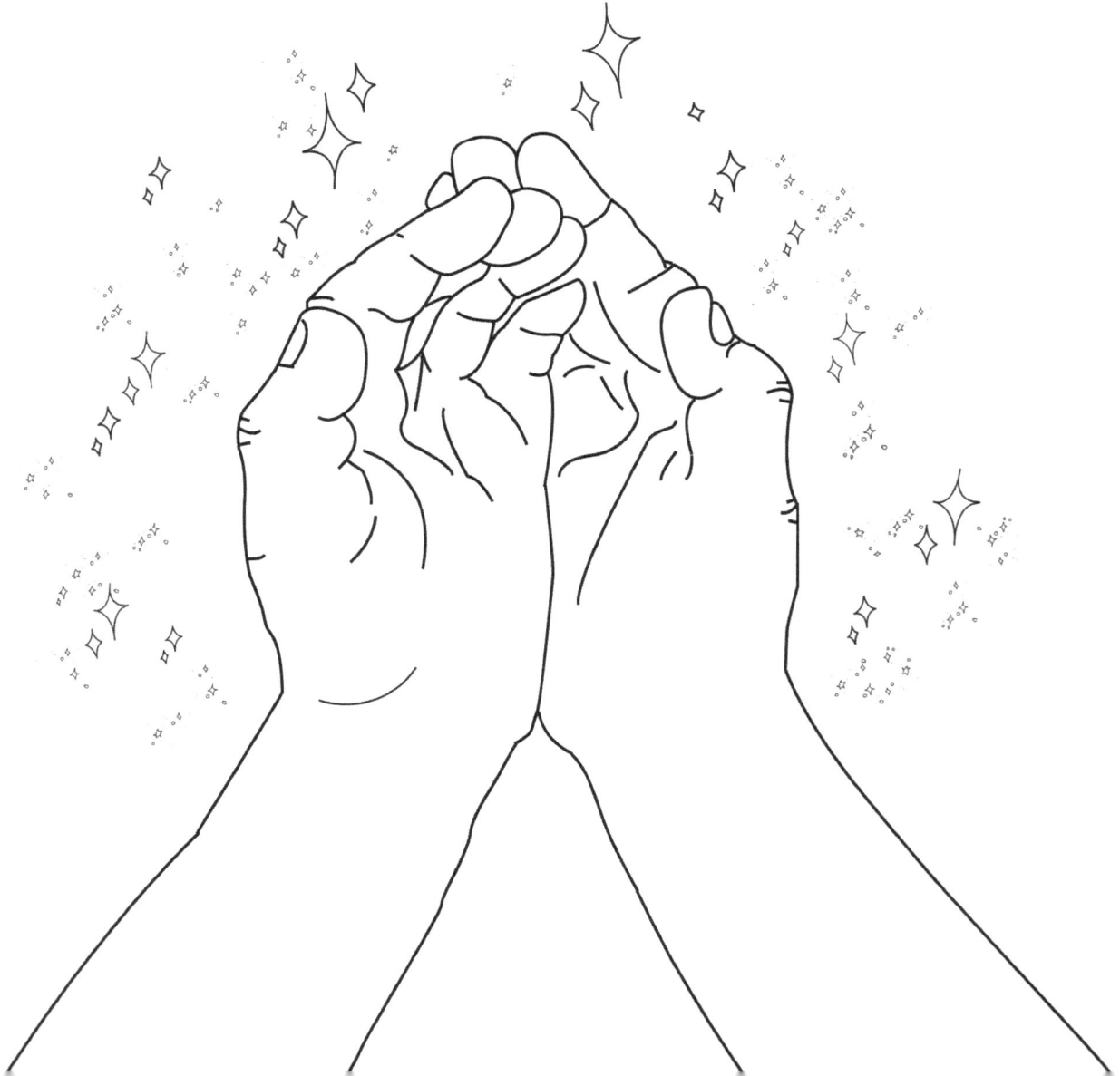

I know I can't see them germs, but I want to stalk 'em.

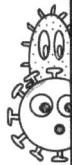

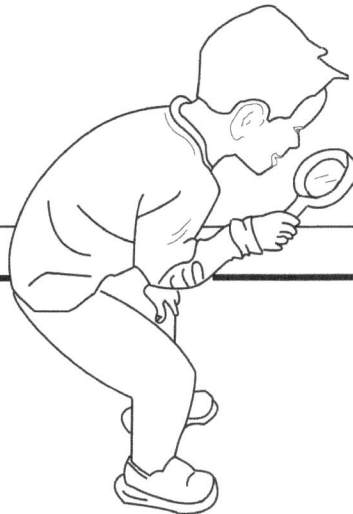

Caution tape round the sink.

I had to destroy 'em!

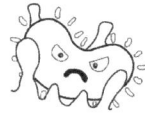
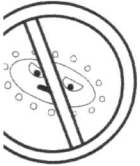
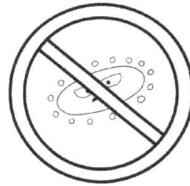
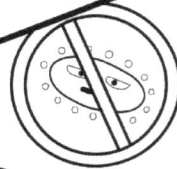
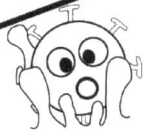

CAUTION

CAUTION

CAUT

CAU

They runnin' from me but
the soap had to hawk 'em
DOWN!

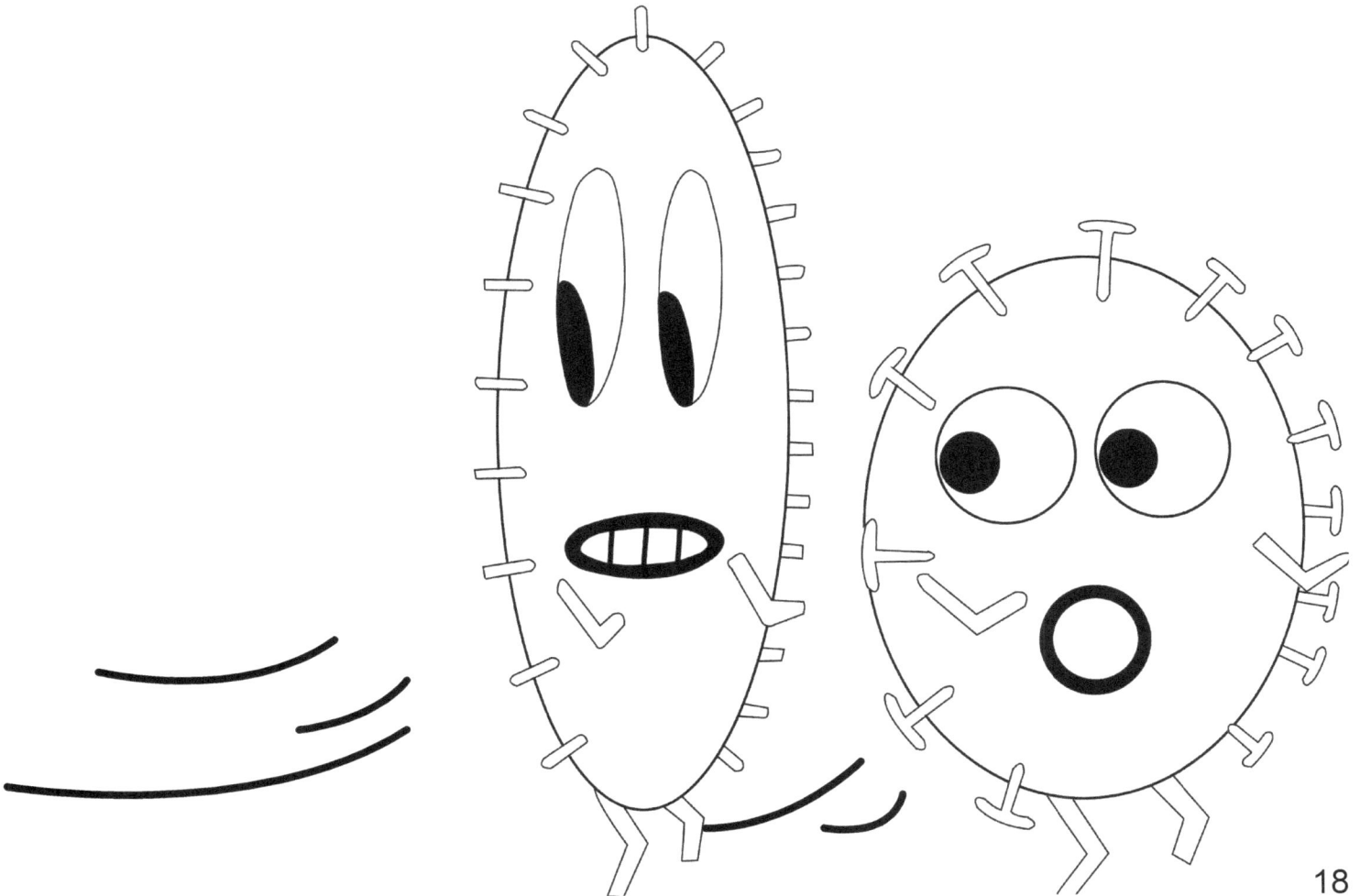

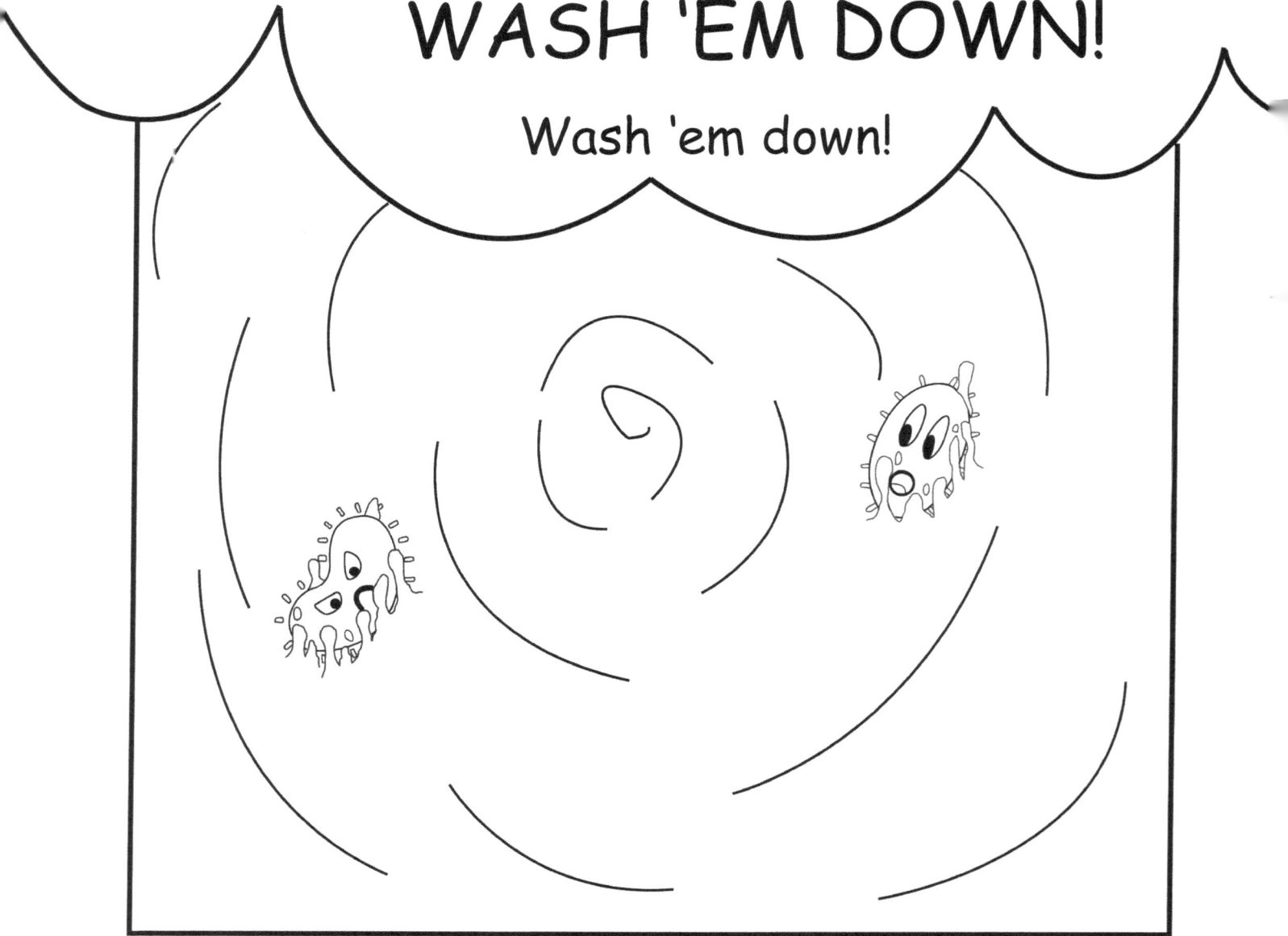

WASH 'EM DOWN!

Wash 'em down!

WASH 'EM DOWN!

Wash 'em down!

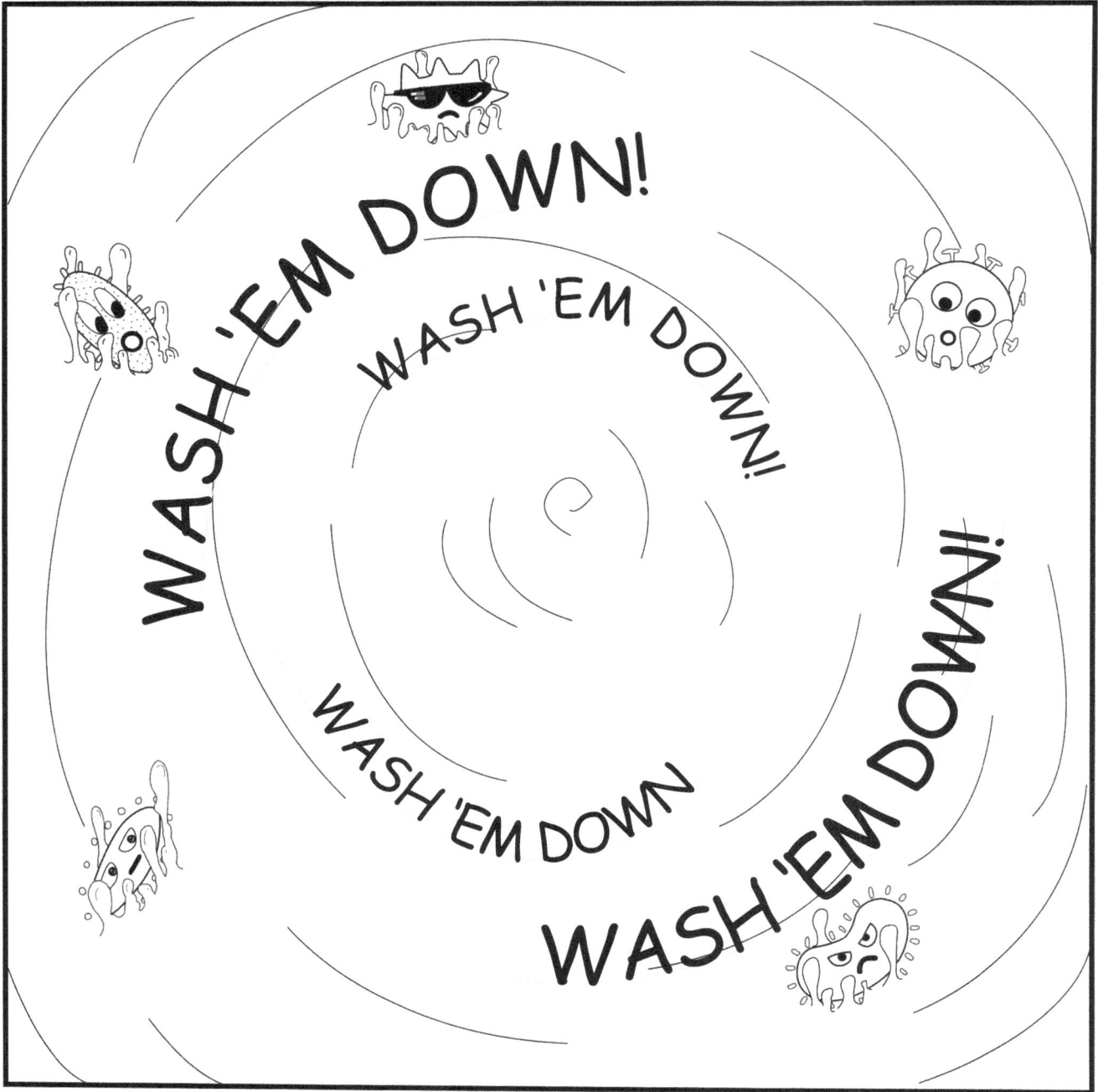

Sparkle and Shine!

Wash your hands every time!

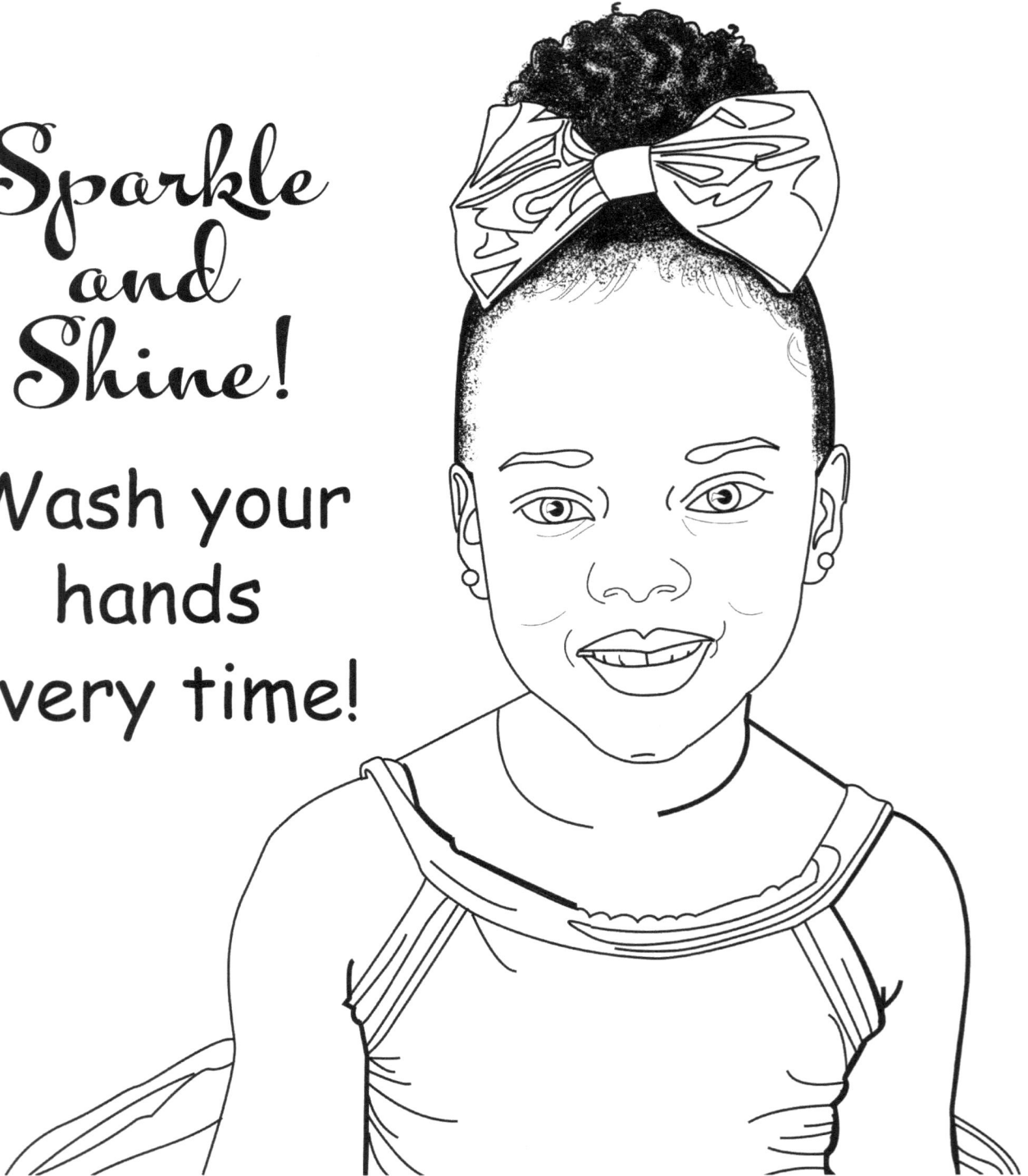

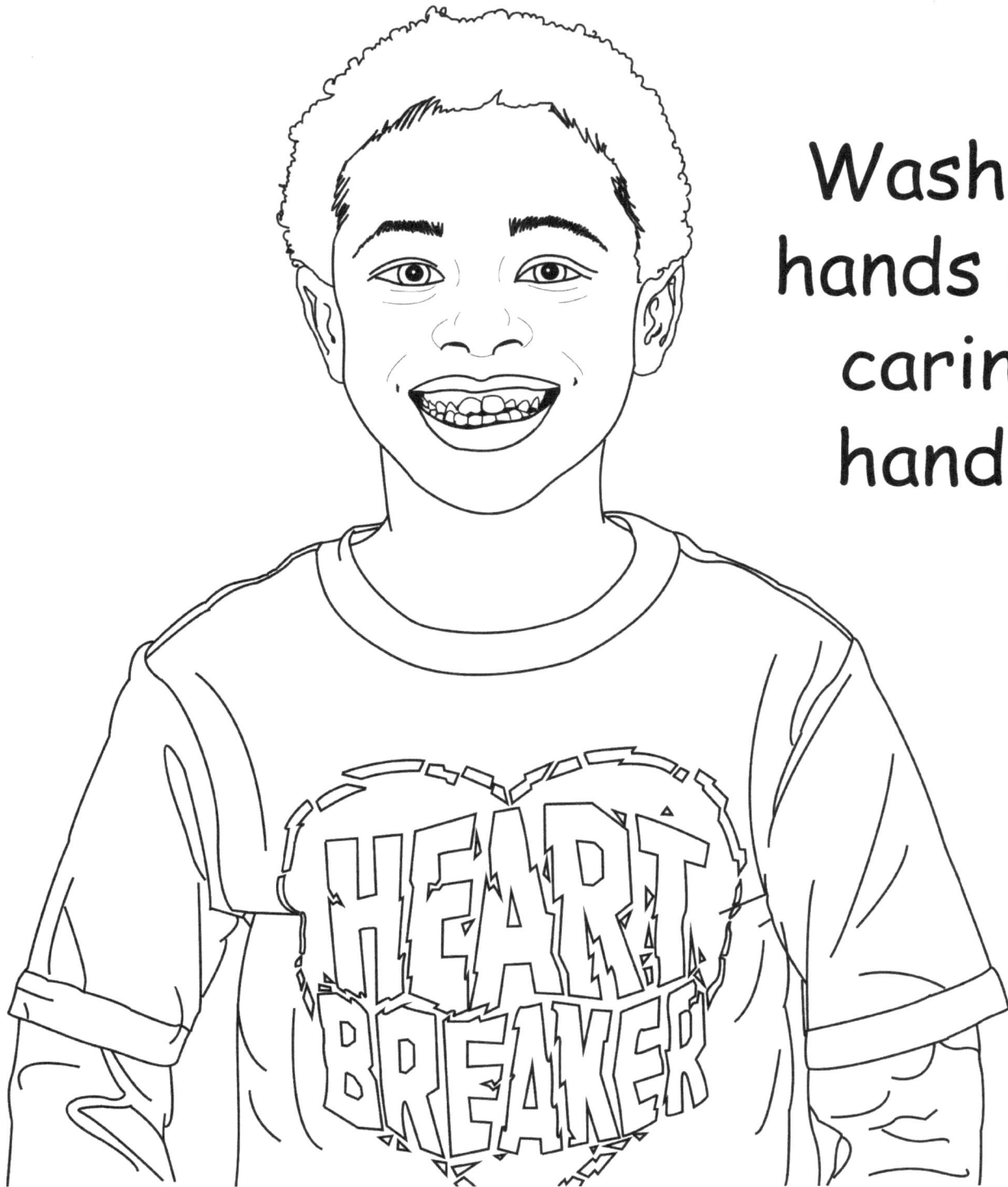

Washed hands are caring hands!

The more you care, the more you wash!

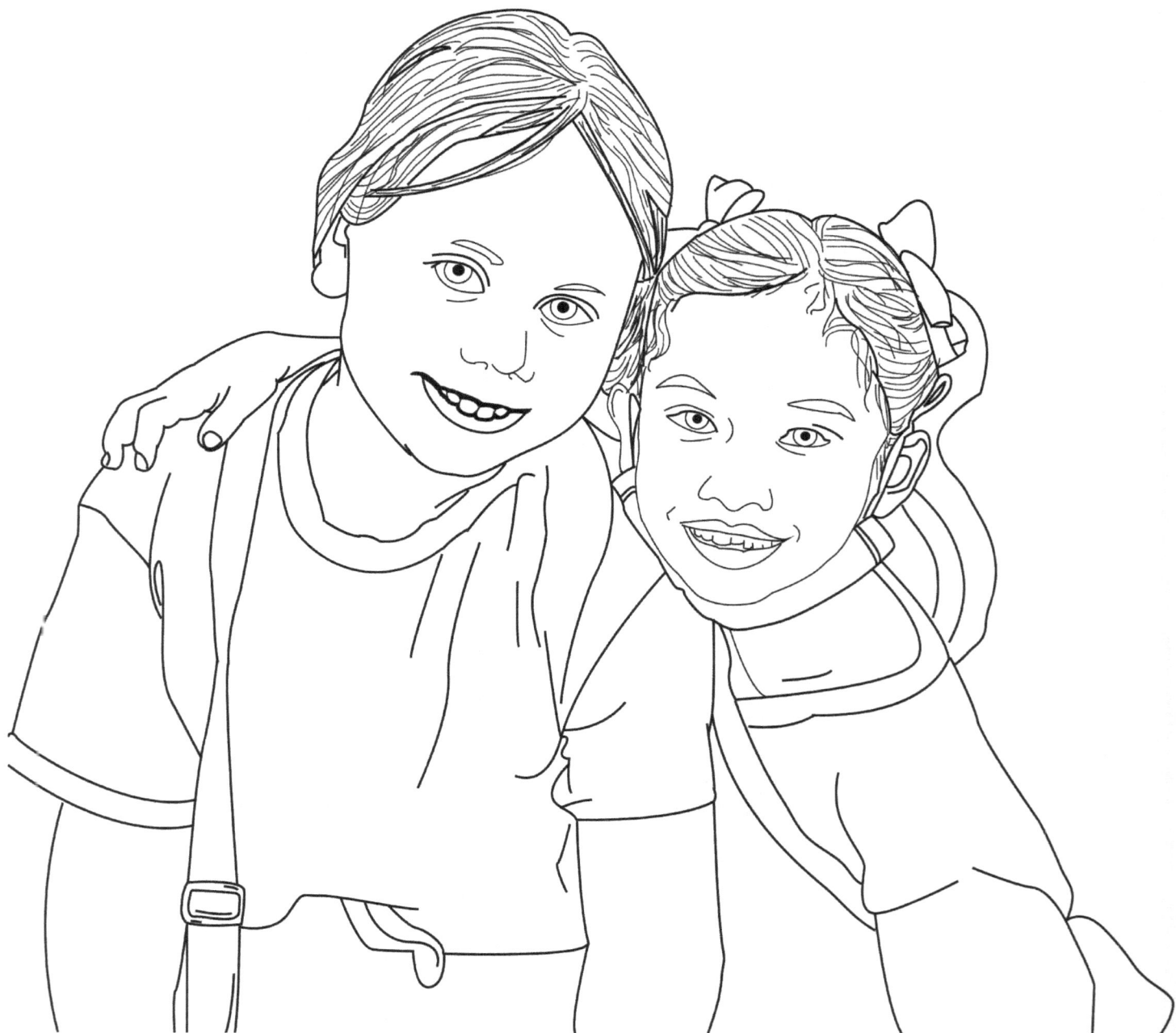

Dedication

I am eternally grateful for all of my "Cool Cats" that I have had the opportunity to stand before and lead. Thank you for being my inspiration and entering the classroom ready to learn each day. I love you all so very much!

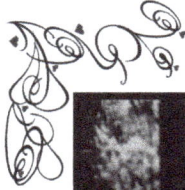

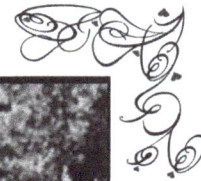

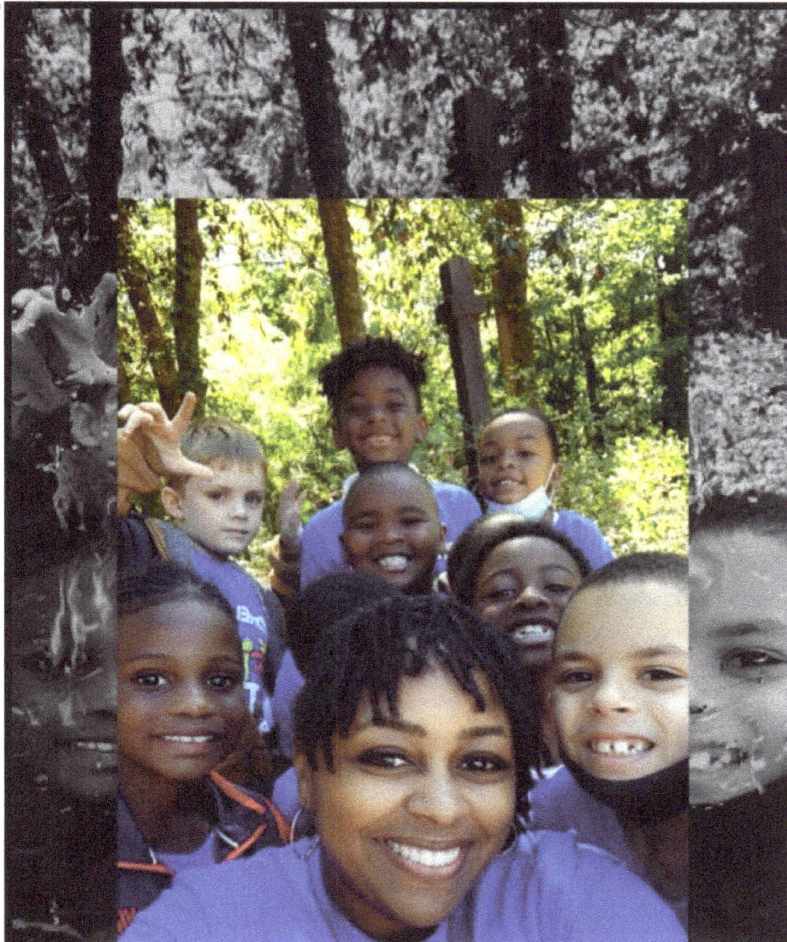

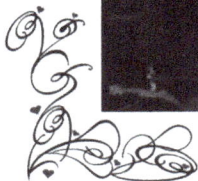

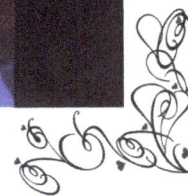

www.ingramcontent.com/pod-product-compliance
Lightning Source LLC
Chambersburg PA
CBHW042348030426

42335CB00031B/3497